Make Your Homemade Hand Sanitizer

An Easy Guide to Make Your Best Homemade Hand Sanitizer with Natural Essential Oils Recipes and Isopropyl Alcohol Content to Kill Viruses.

Written by

Olivia Holliver

Disclaimer Notice:

Please note the information contained within this document is for educational and entertainment purposes only. All effort has been executed to present accurate, up to date, and reliable, complete information. No warranties of any kind are declared or implied. Readers acknowledge that the author is not engaging in the rendering of legal, financial, medical or professional advice. The content within this book has been derived from various sources. Please consult a licensed professional before attempting any techniques outlined in this book.

By reading this document, the reader agrees that under no circumstances is the author responsible for any losses, direct or indirect, which are incurred as a result of the use of information contained within this document, including, but not limited to, — errors, omissions, or inaccuracies.

Table of Contents

Introduction and Basics

Hand sanitizers are the need of the hour, as every year comes with a new set of viral epidemics, they are important to prevent them from spreading. In such scenarios, personal hygiene is of utmost importance, and hand sanitizers are a certified method of keeping the hands free from germs. A person cannot wash his hands all the time; however, he can easily use these gel-like liquids to reduce the germs on his hands. Kids, especially, can be made to use these sanitizers to keep their hands clean before eating anything.

Hand sanitizers come in different varieties and forms. Usually, they are available in a gel like consistency; however, they are also available in lotions, liquid sprays, and foams like consistency.

Commercially, hand sanitizers are made using some percent of alcohol mixed with rubbing alcohol (Isopropyl alcohol) and ethanol. Where those are the basic germ reducing ingredients of these sanitizers, other ingredients are also added to the liquid to add certain fragrance and color to the sanitizer. Triclosan is another commonly used chemical that is added to hand sanitizers to kill some strains of bacteria.

Since there are several commercially produced hand sanitizers available in the market, it is difficult to recognize the ones with good quality. At times people don't feel comfortable using a hand sanitizer, which is filled with added chemicals. Those chemicals can be harmful to sensitive skin as well. For instance, triclosan was recently banned in 2016 by USA FDA for its use in antibacterial soap. It was later banned even for the hand washes. As the debate on the use of triclosan still goes on, many companies are using the chemical without any health concern.

Thus, commercially produced hand sanitizers cannot be trusted, and it is advisable to make your own hand sanitizer at home. By using quality products, and making smart choices, these hand sanitizers can be efficiently made without costing much. Especially, during the season of cold, flu and COVID-19, when the hand sanitizers are usually sold out or become expensive, the homemade sanitizers can prove to be a great relief.

Homemade sanitizers are essentially different from the commercial ones, as they are prepared with fine quality products, and the recipe can be customized to add scents of your choice. Instead of using harmful chemicals, the homemade recipe calls for ingredients that are suitable for all the skin types. If a person's skin is sensitive to certain ingredients, he can customize the sanitizer recipe accordingly.

The hand sanitizer recipes shared in this book provide a range of options to people having different skin types and scent preferences. These recipes are particularly designed to fight back the fast-spreading corona virus and its harmful effects. Remember, the basic proportion of alcohol content in a hand sanitizer remains to be sixty percent. The different recipes of hand sanitizers shared in this book make use of that basic formula and drive multiple varieties that will suit everyone's daily routine and work lives. Essential oils are added to give these sanitizers more benefits for the skin. Let's step forward, and try these budget-friendly, chemical-free hand sanitizers and achieve better hygiene for yourself and your family.

Homemade Sanitizer Recipes

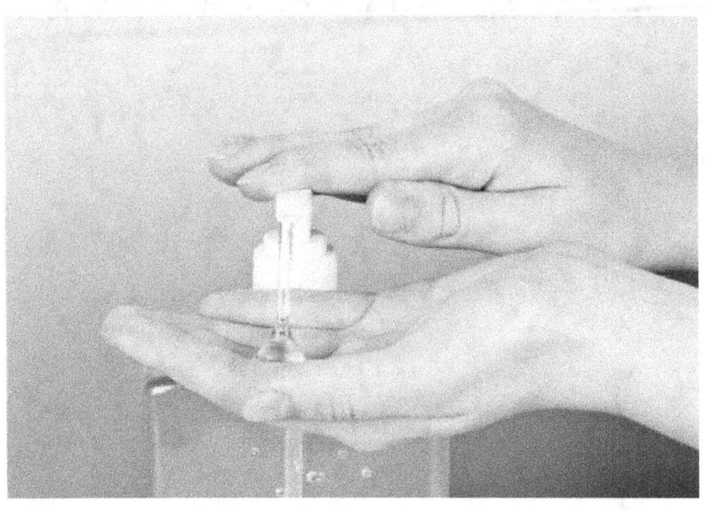

Simple Sanitizer

Ingredients:

- 2/3 cup rubbing alcohol
- 1/3 cup aloe vera gel

Instructions:

1. In a glass bowl, add the rubbing alcohol and aloe vera gel and mix until well combined.

2. Through a funnel, pour the hand sanitizer
   into small, clean squirt bottles.

3. Store in a cool place out of direct sunlight.

4. Remember to shake gently before each use.

Destroyer Essential Oil Sanitizer

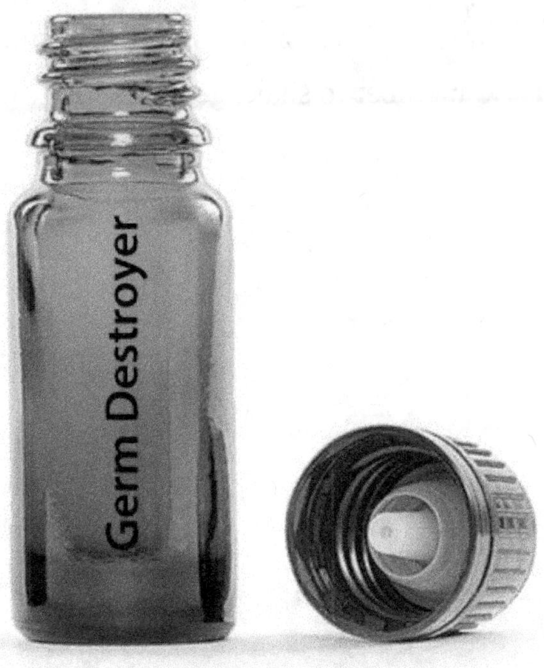

Ingredients:

- 20 drops germ destroyer essential oil
- ¼ cup aloe vera gel

Instructions:

1. In a glass bowl, add the essential oil and aloe vera gel and mix until well combined.

2. Through a funnel, pour the hand sanitizer into small, clean squirt bottles.

3. Store in a cool place out of direct sunlight.

4. Remember to shake gently before each use.

Eucalyptus Oil Sanitizer

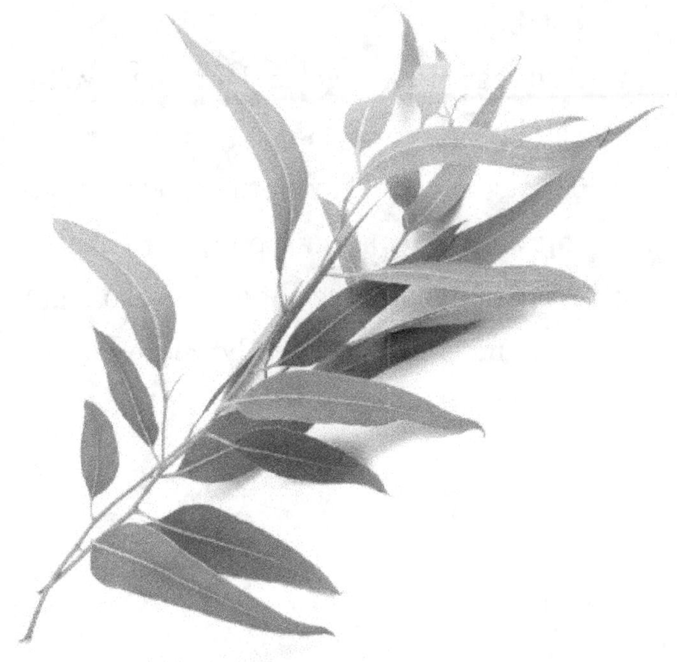

Ingredients:

- 2/3 cup rubbing alcohol
- 10 drops eucalyptus essential oil
- 1/3 cup aloe vera gel

Instructions:

1. In a glass bowl, add the rubbing alcohol and lemongrass essential oil and stir to combine.
2. Add the aloe vera gel and mix until well combined.
3. Through a funnel, pour the hand sanitizer into small, clean squirt bottles.
4. Store in a cool place out of direct sunlight.
5. Remember to shake gently before each use.

Chamomile Oil Sanitizer

Ingredients:

- 15 drops chamomile essential oil
- 5 drops tea tree oil
- 1 tablespoon rubbing alcohol
- ½ tablespoon aloe vera gel
- 2 cups filtered water

Instructions:

1. In a glass bowl, add the essential oil, tree oil and rubbing alcohol and stir to combine.
2. Add the aloe vera gel and mix until well combined.
3. Now, add the water and mix until well combined.
4. Through a funnel, pour the hand sanitizer into small, clean squirt bottles.
5. Store in a cool place out of direct sunlight.
6. Remember to shake gently before each use.

Peppermint Oil Sanitizer

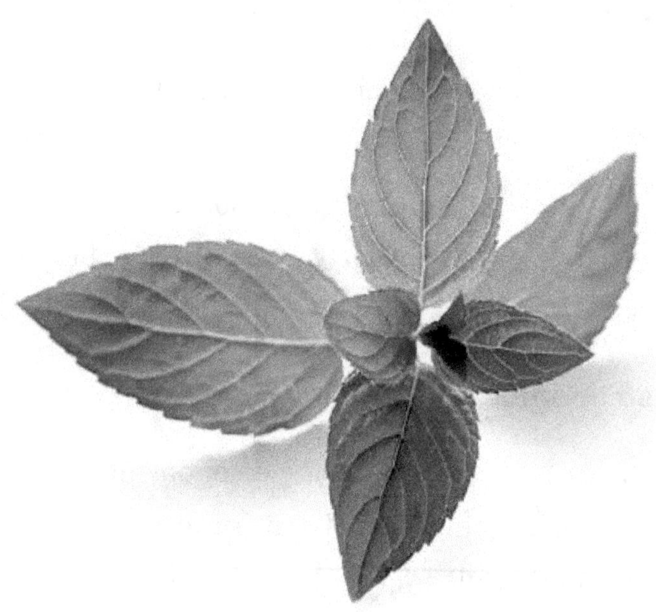

Ingredients:

- 15 drops peppermint essential oil
- 5 drops tea tree oil
- 1 tablespoon rubbing alcohol
- ½ tablespoon aloe vera gel
- 2 cups distilled water

Instructions:

1. In a glass bowl, add the essential oil, tree oil and rubbing alcohol and stir to combine.
2. Add the aloe vera gel and mix until well combined.
3. Now, add the water and mix until well combined.
4. Through a funnel, pour the hand sanitizer into small, clean squirt bottles.
5. Store in a cool place out of direct sunlight.
6. Remember to shake gently before each use.

Lavender Oil Sanitizer

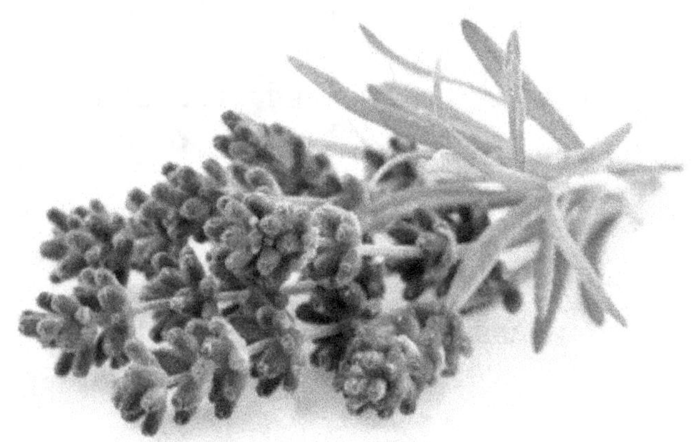

Ingredients:

- 8-10 drops lavender essential oil
- 2/3 cup rubbing alcohol
- 1/3 cup pure aloe vera gel

Instructions:

1. In a glass bowl, add the essential oil and rubbing alcohol and stir to combine.

2. Add the aloe vera gel and mix until well combined.

3. Through a funnel, pour the hand sanitizer into small, clean squirt bottles.

4. Store in a cool place out of direct sunlight.

5. Remember to shake gently before each use.

Lavender & Tea Tree Oil Sanitizer

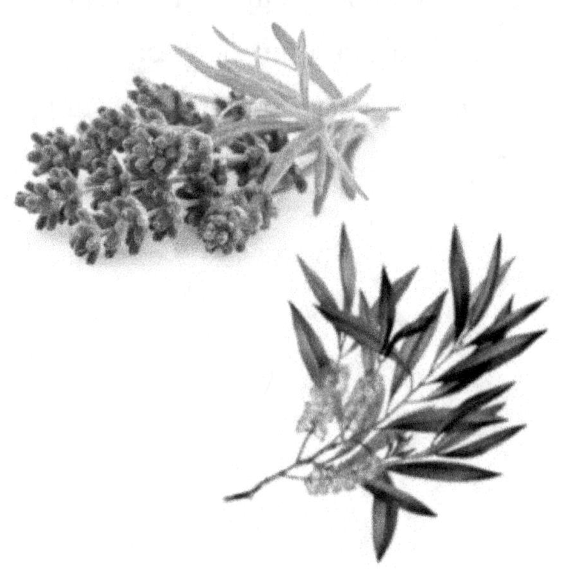

Ingredients:

- 20 drops lavender essential oil

- 5 drops tea tree oil

- 2 tablespoons rubbing alcohol

- ½ tablespoons aloe vera gel

- 2 cups filtered water

Instructions:

6. In a glass bowl, add the essential oil, tree oil and rubbing alcohol and stir to combine.

7. Add the aloe vera gel and mix until well combined.

8. Now, add the water and mix until well combined.

9. Through a funnel, pour the hand sanitizer into small, clean squirt bottles.

10. Store in a cool place out of direct sunlight.

11. Remember to shake gently before each use.

Lemongrass & Cinnamon Oil Sanitizer

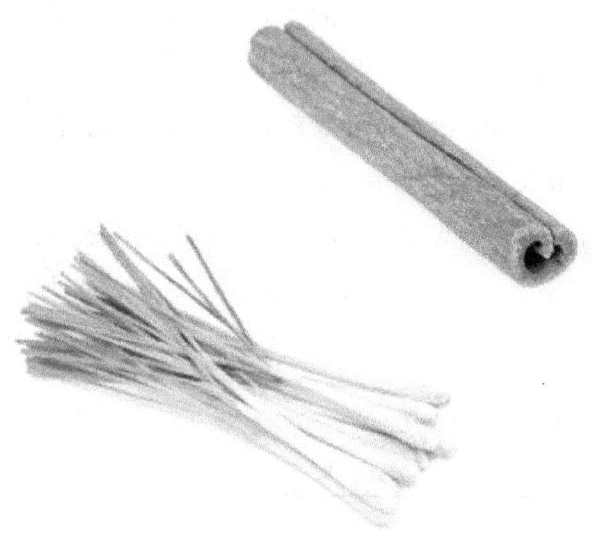

Ingredients:

- ¼ cup aloe vera gel
- ½ teaspoon vegetable glycerin
- 1 tablespoon rubbing alcohol
- 5 drops lemongrass essential oil
- 10 drops cinnamon essential oil

- 10 drops tea tree oil

Lemon Oil Sanitizer

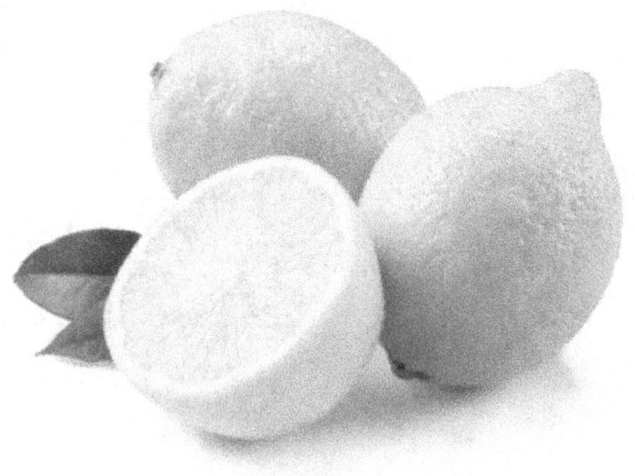

Ingredients:

- 5 drops lemon essential oil
- 5 drops tea tree oil
- 1 tablespoon rubbing alcohol
- ½ tablespoons aloe vera gel
- 2 cups filtered water

Instructions:

1. In a glass bowl, add the essential oil, tree oil and rubbing alcohol and stir to combine.
2. Add the aloe vera gel and mix until well combined.
3. Now, add the water and mix until well combined.
4. Through a funnel, pour the hand sanitizer into small, clean squirt bottles.
5. Store in a cool place out of direct sunlight.
6. Remember to shake gently before each use.

Orange Oil Sanitizer

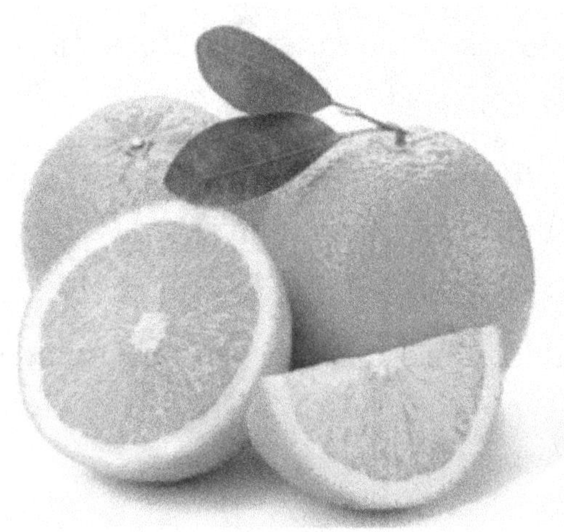

Ingredients:

- 5 drops orange essential oil
- 5 drops tea tree oil
- 1 tablespoon rubbing alcohol
- ½ tablespoons aloe vera gel
- 2 cups filtered water

Instructions:

7. In a glass bowl, add the essential oil, tree oil and rubbing alcohol and stir to combine.

8. Add the aloe vera gel and mix until well combined.

9. Now, add the water and mix until well combined.

10. Through a funnel, pour the hand sanitizer into small, clean squirt bottles.

11. Store in a cool place out of direct sunlight.

12. Remember to shake gently before each use.

Cinnamon Oil Sanitizer

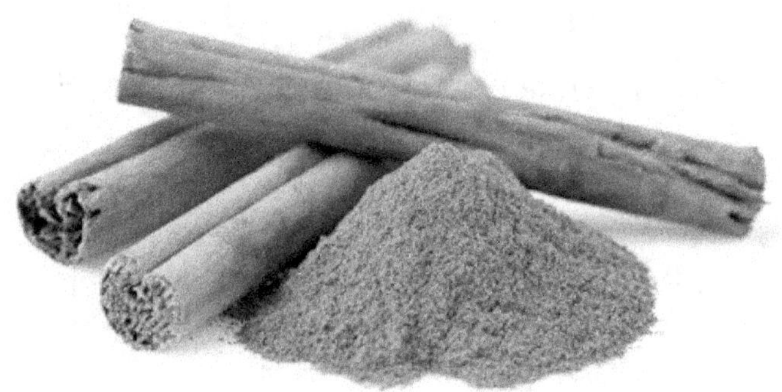

Ingredients:

- 5 drops cinnamon essential oil
- 5 drops tea tree oil
- 1 tablespoon rubbing alcohol
- ½ tablespoons aloe vera gel
- 2 cups filtered swater

Instructions:

1. In a glass bowl, add the essential oil, tree oil and rubbing alcohol and stir to combine.

2. Add the aloe vera gel and mix until well combined.

3. Now, add the water and mix until well combined.

4. Through a funnel, pour the hand sanitizer into small, clean squirt bottles.

5. Store in a cool place out of direct sunlight.

6. Remember to shake gently before each use.

Cardamom Oil Sanitizer

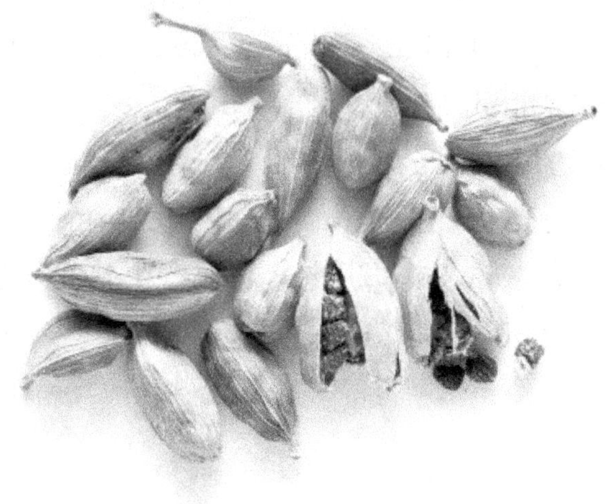

Ingredients:

- 15 drops cardamom essential oil
- 5 drops tea tree oil
- 1 tablespoon rubbing alcohol
- ½ tablespoons aloe vera gel
- 2 cups filtered water

Instructions:

1. In a glass bowl, add the essential oil, tree oil and rubbing alcohol and stir to combine.

2. Add the aloe vera gel and mix until well combined.

3. Now, add the water and mix until well combined.

4. Through a funnel, pour the hand sanitizer into small, clean squirt bottles.

5. Store in a cool place out of direct sunlight.

6. Remember to shake gently before each use.

Clove Oil Sanitizer

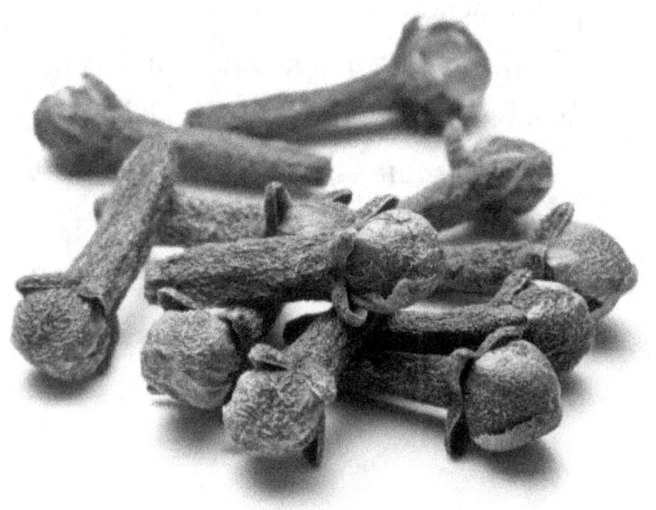

Ingredients:

- 20 drops clove essential oil
- 5 drops tea tree oil
- 2 tablespoons rubbing alcohol
- ½ tablespoons aloe vera gel
- 2 cups filtered water

Instructions:

1. In a glass bowl, add the essential oil, tree oil and rubbing alcohol and stir to combine.
2. Add the aloe vera gel and mix until well combined.
3. Now, add the water and mix until well combined.
4. Through a funnel, pour the hand sanitizer into small, clean squirt bottles.
5. Store in a cool place out of direct sunlight.
6. Remember to shake gently before each use.

Anise Oil Sanitizer

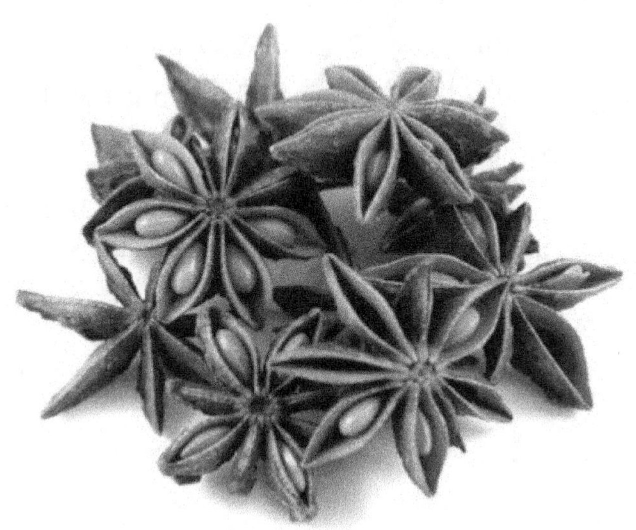

Ingredients:

- 5 drops anise essential oil
- 5 drops tea tree oil
- 1 tablespoon rubbing alcohol
- ½ tablespoons aloe vera gel
- 2 cups filtered water

Instructions:

1. In a glass bowl, add the essential oil, tree oil and rubbing alcohol and stir to combine.

2. Add the aloe vera gel and mix until well combined.

3. Now, add the water and mix until well combined.

4. Through a funnel, pour the hand sanitizer into small, clean squirt bottles.

5. Store in a cool place out of direct sunlight.

6. Remember to shake gently before each use.

Caraway Oil Sanitizer

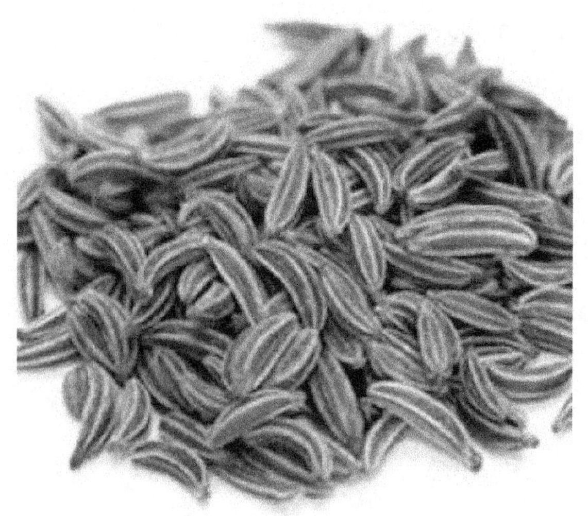

Ingredients:

- 5 drops caraway essential oil
- 5 drops tea tree oil
- 1 tablespoon rubbing alcohol
- ½ tablespoons aloe vera gel
- 2 cups filtered water

Instructions:

1. In a glass bowl, add the essential oil, tree oil and rubbing alcohol and stir to combine.
2. Add the aloe vera gel and mix until well combined.
3. Now, add the water and mix until well combined.
4. Through a funnel, pour the hand sanitizer into small, clean squirt bottles.
5. Store in a cool place out of direct sunlight.
6. Remember to shake gently before each use.

Orange & Cinnamon Oil Sanitizer

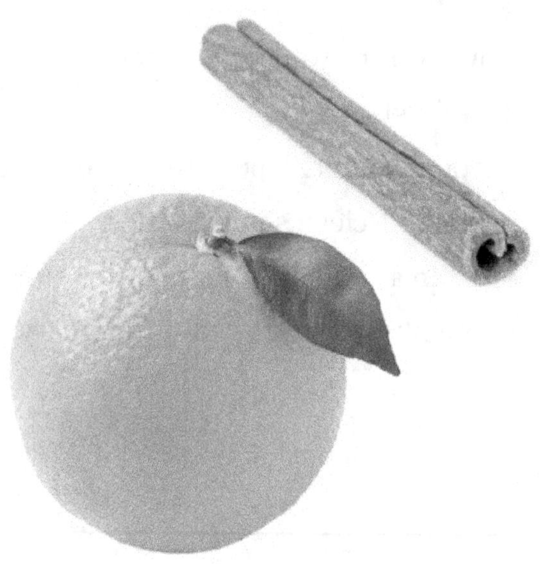

Ingredients:

- 10 drops cinnamon essential oil

- 10 drops sweet orange oil

- ¾ cup rubbing alcohol

- ¼ cup aloe vera gel

- 1/8 cup vegetable glycerin

- 2 cups filtered water

Instructions:

1. In a glass bowl, add the essential oil, orange oil and rubbing alcohol and stir to combine.
2. Add the aloe vera gel and vegetable glycerin and mix until well combined.
3. Now, add the water and mix until well combined.
4. Through a funnel, pour the hand sanitizer into small, clean squirt bottles.
5. Store in a cool place out of direct sunlight.
6. Remember to shake gently before each use.

Fir Needle Oil Sanitizer

Ingredients:

- 15 drops fir needle essential oil
- 5 drops tea tree oil
- 1 tablespoon rubbing alcohol
- ½ tablespoons aloe vera gel
- 2 cups filtered water

Instructions:

1. In a glass bowl, add the essential oil, tree oil and rubbing alcohol and stir to combine.

2. Add the aloe vera gel and mix until well combined.

3. Now, add the water and mix until well combined.

4. Through a funnel, pour the hand sanitizer into small, clean squirt bottles.

5. Store in a cool place out of direct sunlight.

6. Remember to shake gently before each use.

Douglas Fir Oil Sanitizer

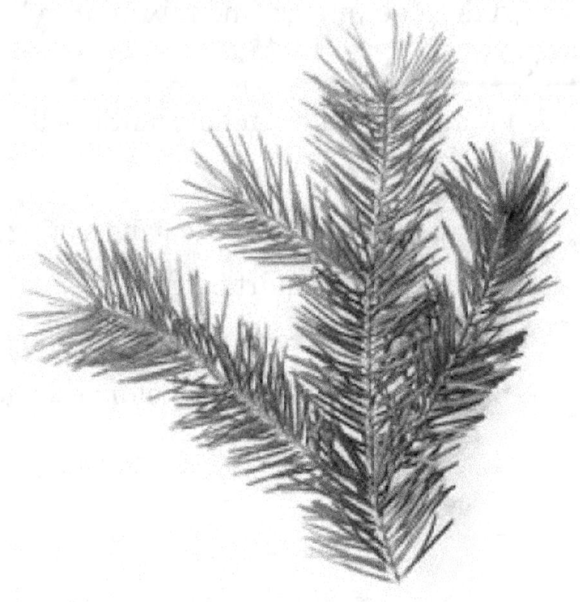

Ingredients:

- 15 drops Douglas fir essential oil
- 5 drops tea tree oil
- 1 tablespoon rubbing alcohol
- ½ tablespoons aloe vera gel
- 2 cups filtered water

Instructions:

1. In a glass bowl, add the essential oil, tree oil and rubbing alcohol and stir to combine.

2. Add the aloe vera gel and mix until well combined.

3. Now, add the water and mix until well combined.

4. Through a funnel, pour the hand sanitizer into small, clean squirt bottles.

5. Store in a cool place out of direct sunlight.

6. Remember to shake gently before each use.

Balsam Fir Oil Sanitizer

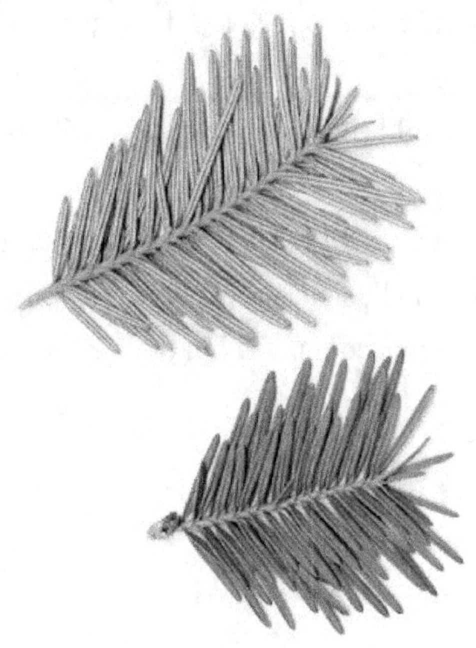

Ingredients:

- 15 drops balsam fir essential oil
- 5 drops tea tree oil
- 1 tablespoon rubbing alcohol
- ½ tablespoons aloe vera gel
- 2 cups filtered water

Instructions:

1. In a glass bowl, add the essential oil, tree oil and rubbing alcohol and stir to combine.
2. Add the aloe vera gel and mix until well combined.
3. Now, add the water and mix until well combined.
4. Through a funnel, pour the hand sanitizer into small, clean squirt bottles.
5. Store in a cool place out of direct sunlight.
6. Remember to shake gently before each use.

Frankincense Oil Sanitizer

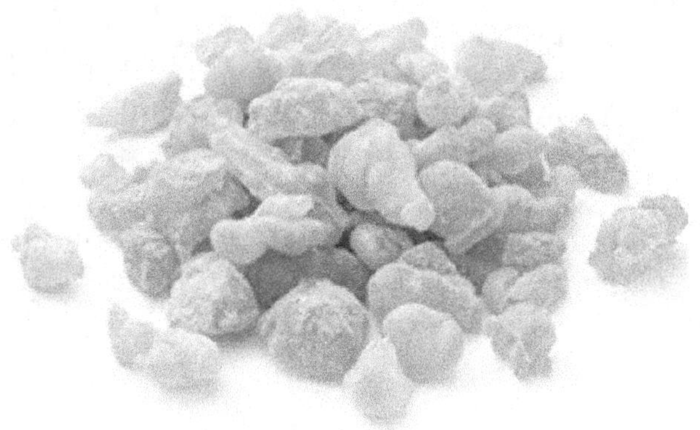

Ingredients:

- 5 drops frankincense essential oil
- 5 drops tea tree oil
- 1 tablespoon rubbing alcohol
- ½ tablespoons aloe vera gel
- 2 cups filtered water

Instructions:

1. In a glass bowl, add the essential oil, tree oil and rubbing alcohol and stir to combine.
2. Add the aloe vera gel and mix until well combined.
3. Now, add the water and mix until well combined.
4. Through a funnel, pour the hand sanitizer into small, clean squirt bottles.
5. Store in a cool place out of direct sunlight.
6. Remember to shake gently before each use.

Vanilla Oil Sanitizer

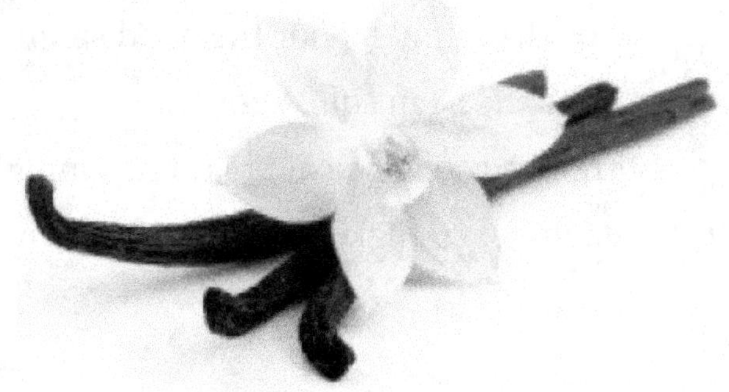

Ingredients:

- 15 drops vanilla essential oil
- 5 drops tea tree oil
- 1 tablespoon rubbing alcohol
- ½ tablespoons aloe vera gel
- 2 cups filtered water

Instructions:

1. In a glass bowl, add the essential oil, tree oil and rubbing alcohol and stir to combine.

2. Add the aloe vera gel and mix until well combined.

3. Now, add the water and mix until well combined.

4. Through a funnel, pour the hand sanitizer into small, clean squirt bottles.

5. Store in a cool place out of direct sunlight.

6. Remember to shake gently before each use.

Eucalyptus Oil Sanitizer

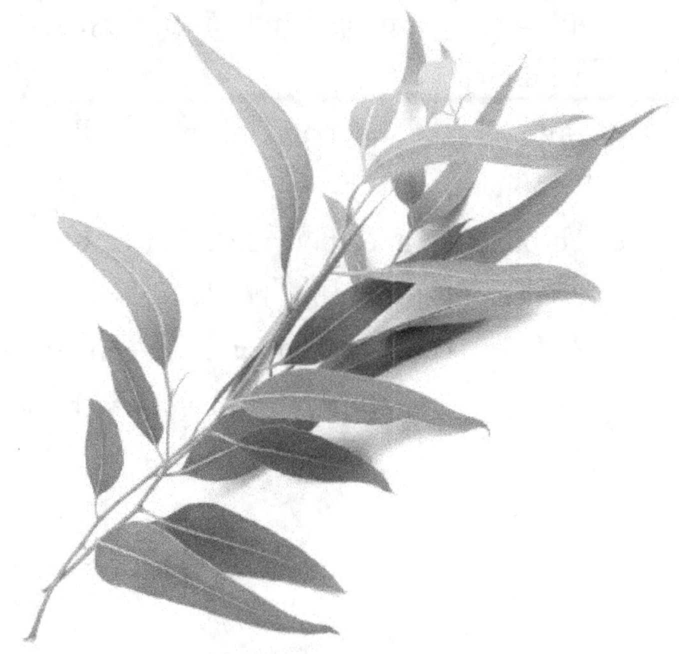

Ingredients:

- 15 drops eucalyptus essential oil
- 5 drops tea tree oil
- 1 tablespoon rubbing alcohol
- ½ tablespoons aloe vera gel
- 2 cups filtered water

Instructions:

1. In a glass bowl, add the essential oil, tree oil and rubbing alcohol and stir to combine.
2. Add the aloe vera gel and mix until well combined.
3. Now, add the water and mix until well combined.
4. Through a funnel, pour the hand sanitizer into small, clean squirt bottles.
5. Store in a cool place out of direct sunlight.
6. Remember to shake gently before each use.

Sandalwood Oil Sanitizer

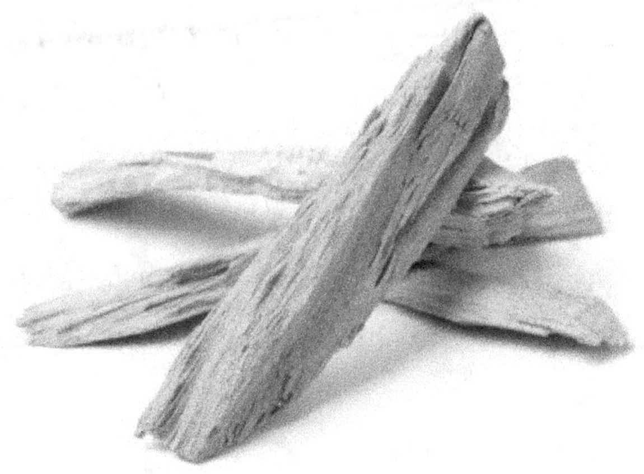

Ingredients:

- 5 drops sandalwood essential oil
- 5 drops tea tree oil
- 1 tablespoon rubbing alcohol
- ½ tablespoons aloe vera gel
- 2 cups filtered water

Instructions:

1. In a glass bowl, add the essential oil, tree oil and rubbing alcohol and stir to combine.
2. Add the aloe vera gel and mix until well combined.
3. Now, add the water and mix until well combined.
4. Through a funnel, pour the hand sanitizer into small, clean squirt bottles.
5. Store in a cool place out of direct sunlight.
6. Remember to shake gently before each use.

Cedarwood Oil Sanitizer

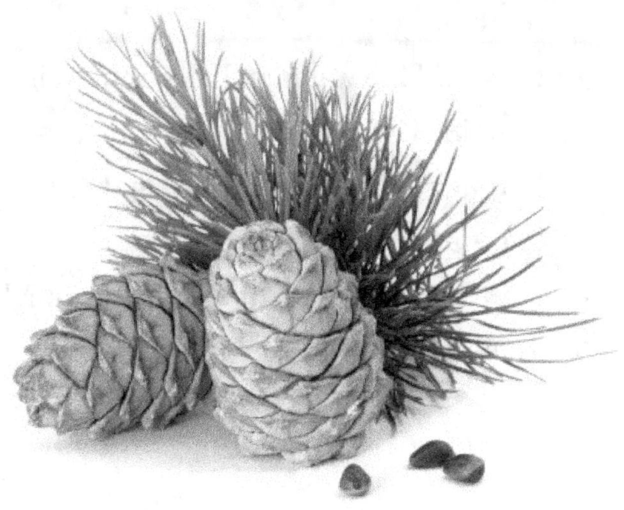

Ingredients:

- 5 drops cedarwood essential oil
- 5 drops tea tree oil
- 1 tablespoon rubbing alcohol
- ½ tablespoons aloe vera gel
- 2 cups filtered water

Instructions:

1. In a glass bowl, add the essential oil, tree oil and rubbing alcohol and stir to combine.
2. Add the aloe vera gel and mix until well combined.
3. Now, add the water and mix until well combined.
4. Through a funnel, pour the hand sanitizer into small, clean squirt bottles.
5. Store in a cool place out of direct sunlight.
6. Remember to shake gently before each use.

Tea Tree Oil Sanitizer

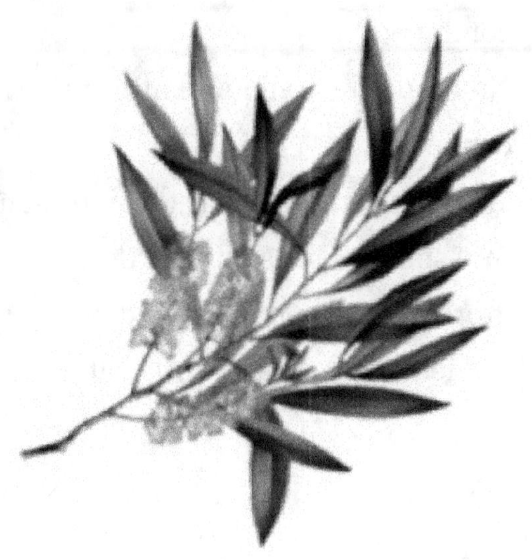

Ingredients:

- 5 drops tea tree essential oil
- 5 drops tea tree oil
- 1 tablespoon rubbing alcohol
- ½ tablespoons aloe vera gel
- 2 cups filtered water

Instructions:

1. In a glass bowl, add the essential oil, tree oil and rubbing alcohol and stir to combine.
2. Add the aloe vera gel and mix until well combined.
3. Now, add the water and mix until well combined.
4. Through a funnel, pour the hand sanitizer into small, clean squirt bottles.
5. Store in a cool place out of direct sunlight.
6. Remember to shake gently before each use.

Vetiver Oil Sanitizer

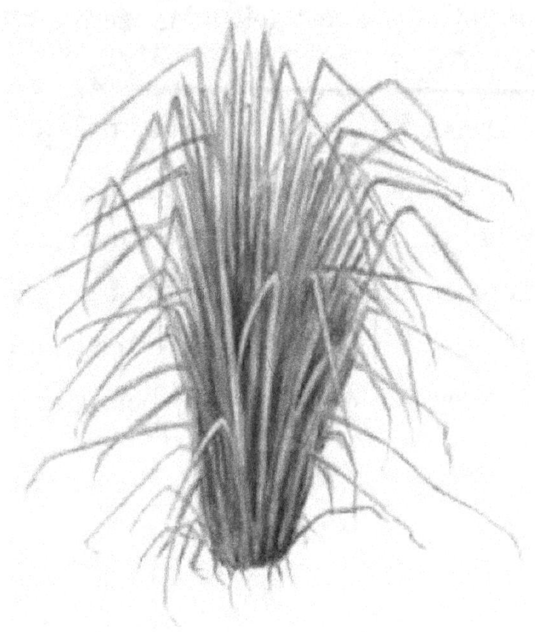

Ingredients:

- 15 drops vetiver essential oil
- 5 drops tea tree oil
- 1 tablespoon rubbing alcohol
- ½ tablespoons aloe vera gel
- 2 cups filtered water

Instructions:

1. In a glass bowl, add the essential oil, tree oil and rubbing alcohol and stir to combine.
2. Add the aloe vera gel and mix until well combined.
3. Now, add the water and mix until well combined.
4. Through a funnel, pour the hand sanitizer into small, clean squirt bottles.
5. Store in a cool place out of direct sunlight.
6. Remember to shake gently before each use.

Ginger Oil Sanitizer

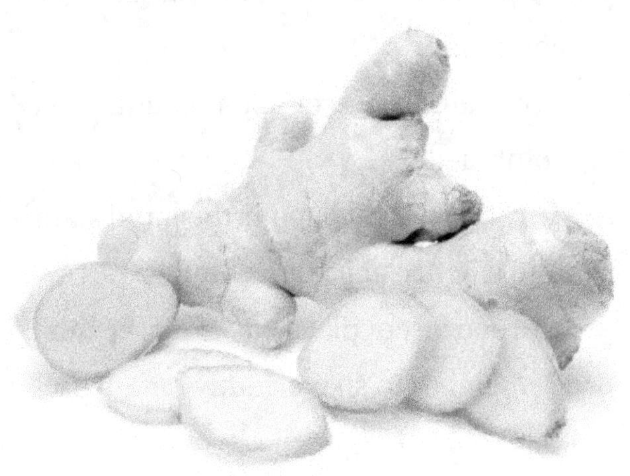

Ingredients:

Ingredients:

- 5 drops ginger essential oil
- 5 drops tea tree oil
- 1 tablespoon rubbing alcohol
- ½ tablespoons aloe vera gel
- 2 cups filtered water

Instructions:

1. In a glass bowl, add the essential oil, tree oil and rubbing alcohol and stir to combine.
2. Add the aloe vera gel and mix until well combined.
3. Now, add the water and mix until well combined.
4. Through a funnel, pour the hand sanitizer into small, clean squirt bottles.
5. Store in a cool place out of direct sunlight.
6. Remember to shake gently before each use.

Rosemary Oil Sanitizer

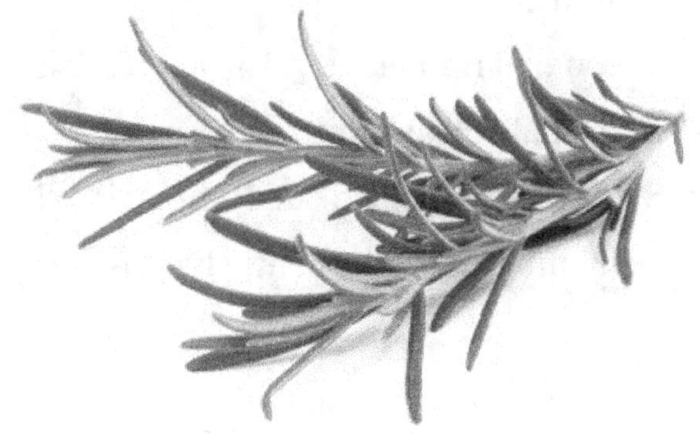

Ingredients:

- 15 drops rosemary essential oil
- 5 drops tea tree oil
- 2 tablespoons rubbing alcohol
- ½ tablespoons aloe vera gel
- 2 cups filtered water

Instructions:

1. In a glass bowl, add the essential oil, tree oil
   and rubbing alcohol and stir to combine.
2. Add the aloe vera gel and mix until well
   combined.
3. Now, add the water and mix until well
   combined.
4. Through a funnel, pour the hand sanitizer
   into small, clean squirt bottles.
5. Store in a cool place out of direct sunlight.
6. Remember to shake gently before each use.

Tarragon Oil Sanitizer

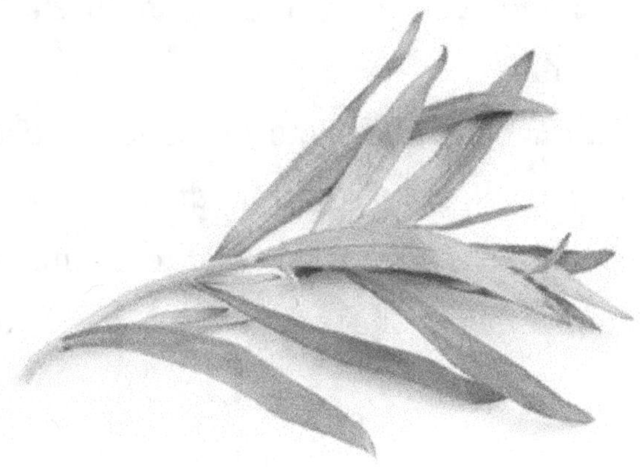

Ingredients:

- 5 drops tarragon essential oil
- 5 drops tea tree oil
- 1 tablespoon rubbing alcohol
- ½ tablespoons aloe vera gel
- 2 cups filtered water

Instructions:

1. In a glass bowl, add the essential oil, tree oil and rubbing alcohol and stir to combine.
2. Add the aloe vera gel and mix until well combined.
3. Now, add the water and mix until well combined.
4. Through a funnel, pour the hand sanitizer into small, clean squirt bottles.
5. Store in a cool place out of direct sunlight.
6. Remember to shake gently before each use.

Orange & Vitamin E Oil Sanitizer

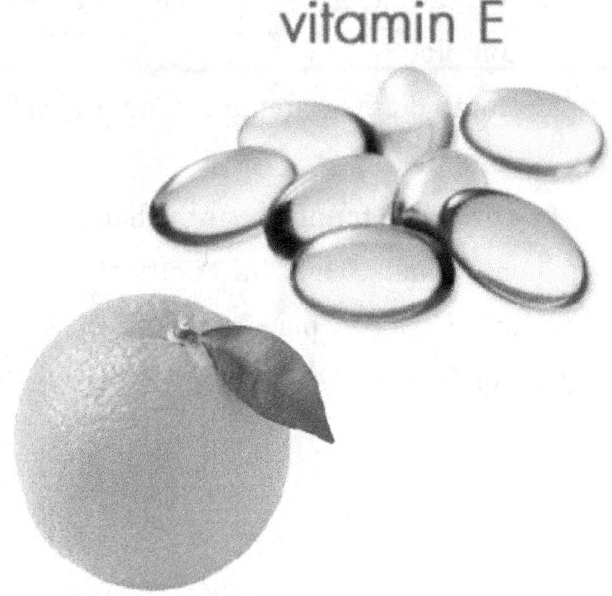

Ingredients:

- 10 drops sweet orange oil
- 2 teaspoons Vitamin E oil
- 1 tablespoon ethyl alcohol
- 2 teaspoons aloe vera gel
- 1 cup filtered water

Instructions:

1. In a glass bowl, add the orange oil, Vitamin E oil and ethyl alcohol and stir to combine.

2. Add the aloe vera gel and mix until well combined.

3. Now, add the water and mix until well combined.

4. Through a funnel, pour the hand sanitizer into small, clean squirt bottles.

5. Store in a cool place out of direct sunlight.

6. Remember to shake gently before each use.

Vitamin E & Lavender Oil Sanitizer

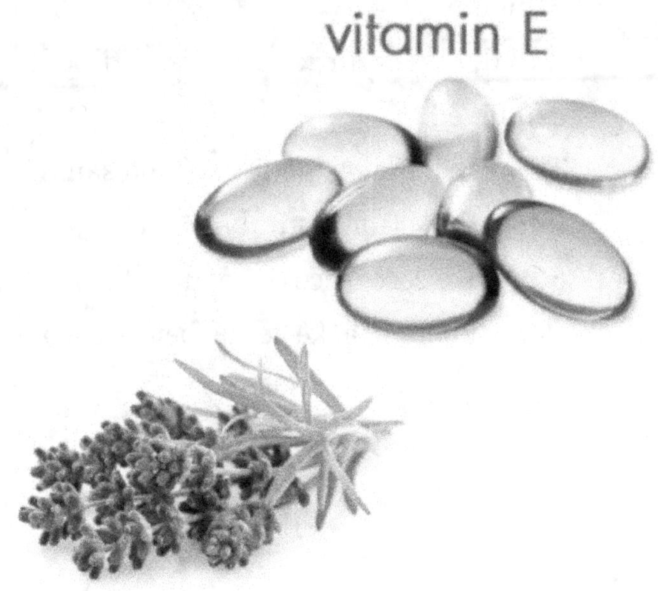

Ingredients:

- 30 drops tea tree essential oil
- 5-10 drops lavender essential oil
- ¼ teaspoon Vitamin E oil
- 3 ounces high-proof vodka
- 1 ounce pure aloe vera gel

Instructions:

1. In a glass bowl, add both essential oils, Vitamin E oil and vodka and stir to combine.
2. Add the aloe vera gel and mix until well combined.
3. Through a funnel, pour the hand sanitizer into small, clean squirt bottles.
4. Store in a cool place out of direct sunlight.
5. Remember to shake gently before each use.

4 Oils & vegetable Glycerin Sanitizer

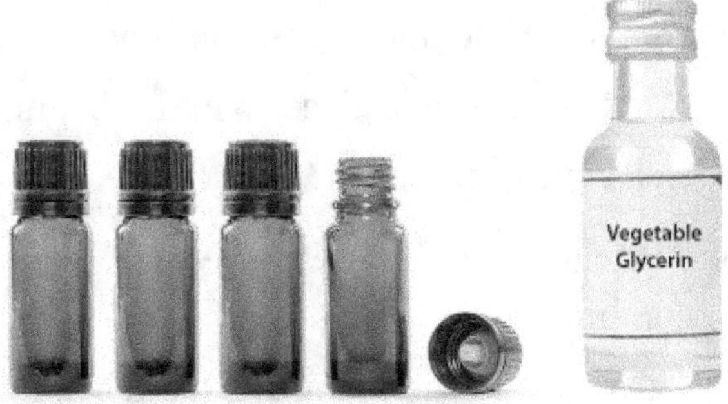

Ingredients:

- 2 drops eucalyptus essential oil
- 2 drops rosemary essential oil
- 2 drops cinnamon leaf essential oil
- 2 drops clove bud essential oil
- 2 tablespoons vodka
- 1 teaspoon aloe vera juice

- ½ teaspoon vegetable glycerin

- 2 tablespoons sterile water

Instructions:

1. In a glass bowl, add all oils, vodka and aloe vera juice and and stir to combine.
2. Add the vegetable glycerin and mix until well combined.
3. Now, add the water and mix until well combined.
4. Through a funnel, pour the hand sanitizer into small, clean squirt bottles.
5. Store in a cool place out of direct sunlight.
6. Remember to shake gently before each use.

Vitamin E Oil Sanitizer

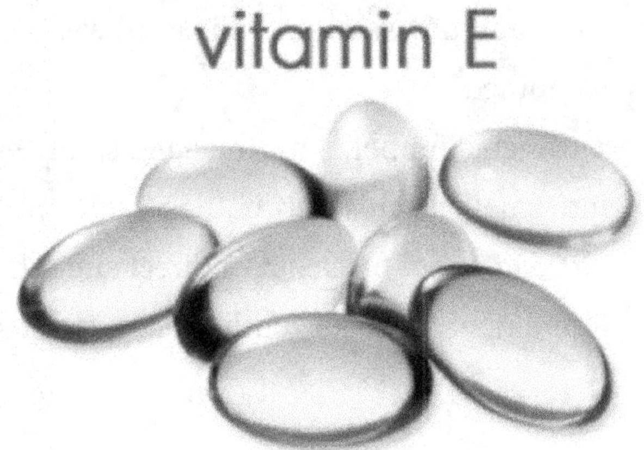

Ingredients:

- 5 drops Vitamin E oil
- 5 drops tea tree oil
- 3 tablespoons aloe vera gel
- 2 cups filtered water

Instructions:

1. In a glass bowl, add the Vitamin E oil and tree oil and stir to combine.

2. Add the aloe vera gel and mix until well combined.

3. Now, add the water and mix until well combined.

4. Through a funnel, pour the hand sanitizer into small, clean squirt bottles.

5. Store in a cool place out of direct sunlight.

6. Remember to shake gently before each use.

5 Oils Sanitizer

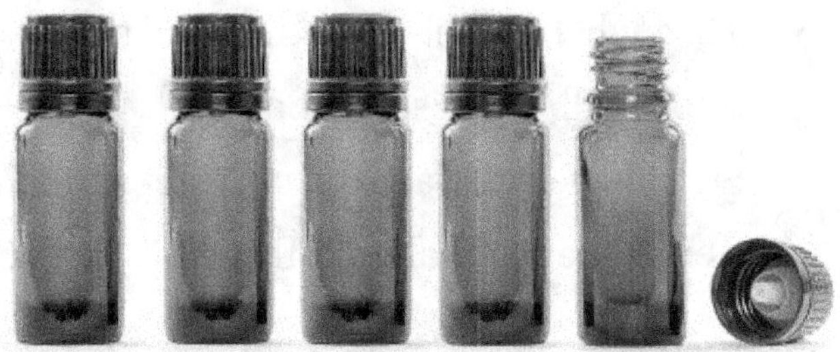

Ingredients:

- 20 drops orange essential oil
- 10 drops lavender essential oil
- 10 drops cinnamon essential oil
- 5 drops rosemary essential oil
- 5 drops clove essential oil
- ¼ cup aloe vera gel

Instructions:

1. In a glass bowl, add all the oils and stir to combine.
2. Add the aloe vera gel and mix until well combined.
3. Through a funnel, pour the hand sanitizer into small, clean squirt bottles.
4. Store in a cool place out of direct sunlight.
5. Remember to shake gently before each use.

4 Oils & Witch Hazel Sanitizer

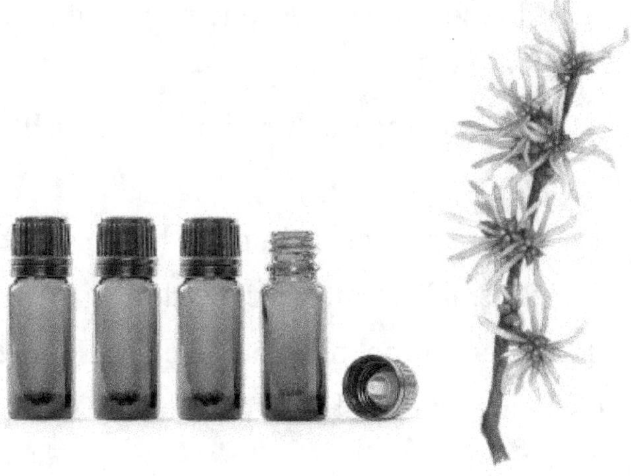

Ingredients:

- 2 teaspoons Vitamin E oil
- 10 drops lavender essential oil
- 10 drops tea tree oil
- 10 drops frankincense oil
- 1 tablespoon witch hazel
- 2 tablespoons aloe vera gel

- 2 cups water

Instructions:

1. In a glass bowl, add all oils and witch hazel and stir to combine.
2. Add the aloe vera gel and mix until well combined.
3. Now, add the water and mix until well combined.
4. Through a funnel, pour the hand sanitizer into small, clean squirt bottles.
5. Store in a cool place out of direct sunlight.
6. Remember to shake gently before each use.

3 Oils & Witch Hazel Sanitizer

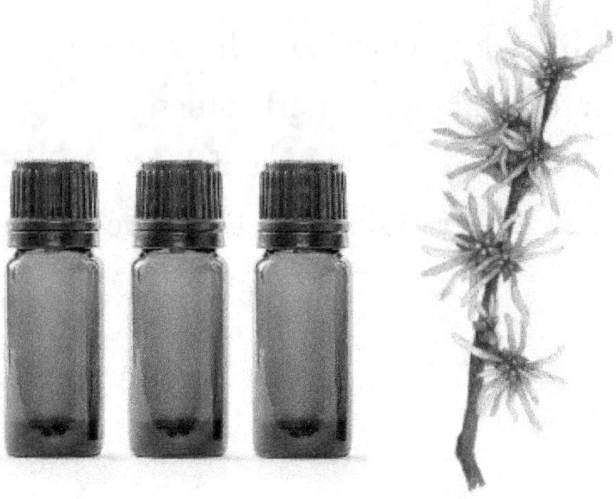

Ingredients:

- 1 teaspoon Vitamin E oil solution
- 10 drops lavender essential oil
- 5 drops lemongrass essential oil
- 4 tablespoons witch hazel
- 2 tablespoons aloe vera gel

Instructions:

1. In a glass bowl, add the Vitamin E oil solution, essential oils and witch hazel and stir to combine.

2. Add the aloe vera gel and mix until well combined.

3. Through a funnel, pour the hand sanitizer into small, clean squirt bottles.

4. Store in a cool place out of direct sunlight.

5. Remember to shake gently before each use.

Aloe Vera Sanitizer

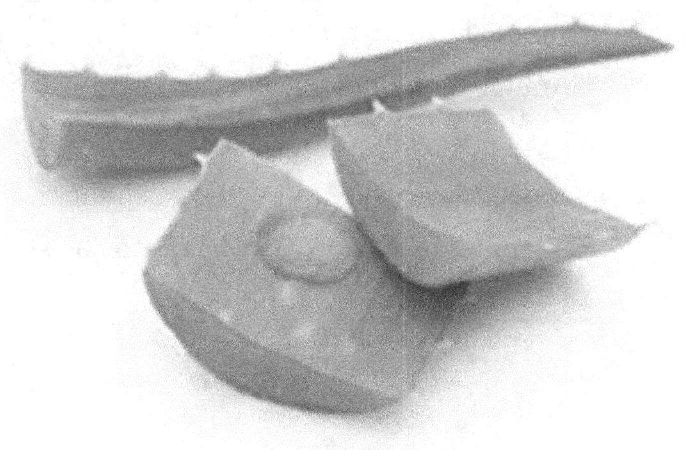

Ingredients:

- ¼ teaspoon Vitamin E oil
- 5 drops lavender essential oil
- 5 drops tea tree oil
- 1 tablespoon hazel extract
- 8 ounces pure aloe vera gel

Instructions:

1. In a glass bowl, add the Vitamin E oil, essential oil, tree oil and hazel extract and stir to combine.
2. Add the aloe vera gel and mix until well combined.
3. Through a funnel, pour the hand sanitizer into small, clean squirt bottles.
4. Store in a cool place out of direct sunlight.
5. Remember to shake gently before each use.

Witch Hazel & Vegetable Glycerin Sanitizer

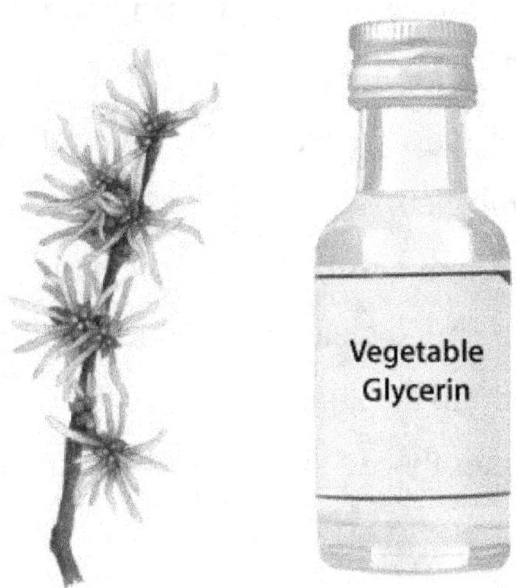

Ingredients:

- 5 drops lemongrass essential oil
- 5 drops rosemary essential oil
- 20 drops tea tree oil
- 2 tablespoons witch hazel
- 1 tablespoon vegetable glycerin

- 2 tablespoons filtered water

Instructions:

1. In a glass bowl, add all oils and witch hazel and stir to combine.
2. Add the vegetable glycerin and mix until well combined.
3. Now, add the water and mix until well combined.
4. Through a funnel, pour the hand sanitizer into small, clean squirt bottles.
5. Store in a cool place out of direct sunlight.
6. Remember to shake gently before each use.

Witch Hazel & Lavender Oil Sanitizer

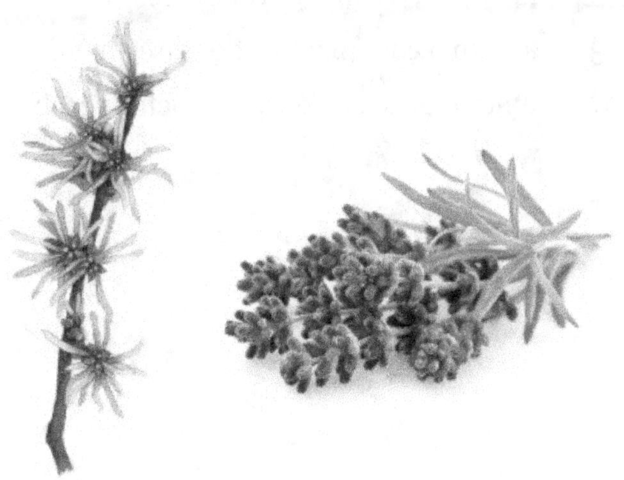

Ingredients:

- ½ cup aloe vera juice
- ¼ cup witch hazel
- 10-20 drops lavender essential oil
- 1 tablespoon organic lavender lotion

Instructions:

1. In a glass bowl, add all the ingredients and mix until well combined.

2. Through a funnel, pour the hand sanitizer into small, clean squirt bottles.

3. Store in a cool place out of direct sunlight.

4. Remember to shake gently before each use.

Water-Free Witch Hazel Sanitizer

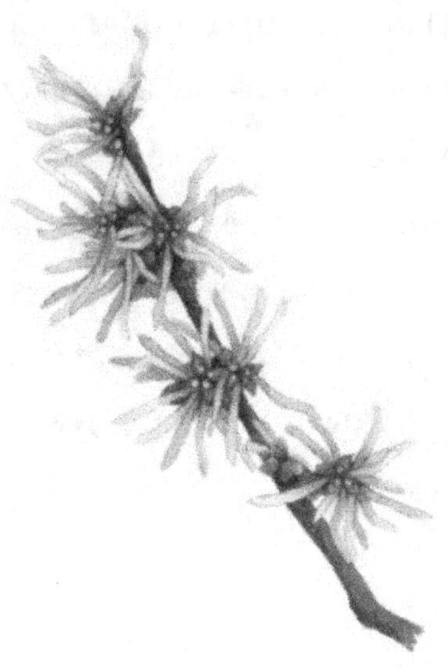

Ingredients:

- 1 teaspoon Vitamin E oil
- 10 drops lavender essential oil
- 6 drops lemongrass essential oil
- 25 drops tea tree oil
- 12 teaspoons witch hazel
- 6 teaspoons aloe vera gel

Instructions:

1. In a glass bowl, add all the oils and witch hazel and stir to combine.
2. Add the aloe vera gel and mix until well combined.
3. Through a funnel, pour the hand sanitizer into small, clean squirt bottles.
4. Store in a cool place out of direct sunlight.
5. Remember to shake gently before each use.

3 Oils & Hazel Extract Sanitizer

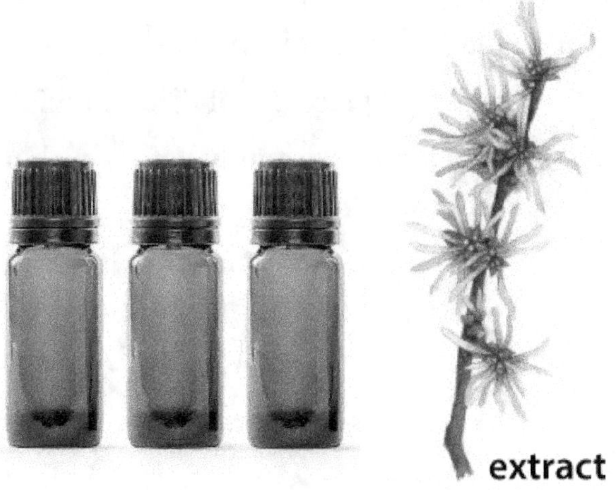

Ingredients:

- 30 drops tea tree essential oil

- 10 drops lavender essential oil

- ¼ teaspoon almond oil

- 1 tablespoon witch hazel extract

- 1 cup aloe vera gel

Instructions:

1. In a glass bowl, add all the oils and witch hazel extract and stir to combine.

2. Add the aloe vera gel and mix until well combined.

3. Through a funnel, pour the hand sanitizer into small, clean squirt bottles.

4. Store in a cool place out of direct sunlight.

5. Remember to shake gently before each use.

Vitamin E Oil & Witch Hazel Sanitizer

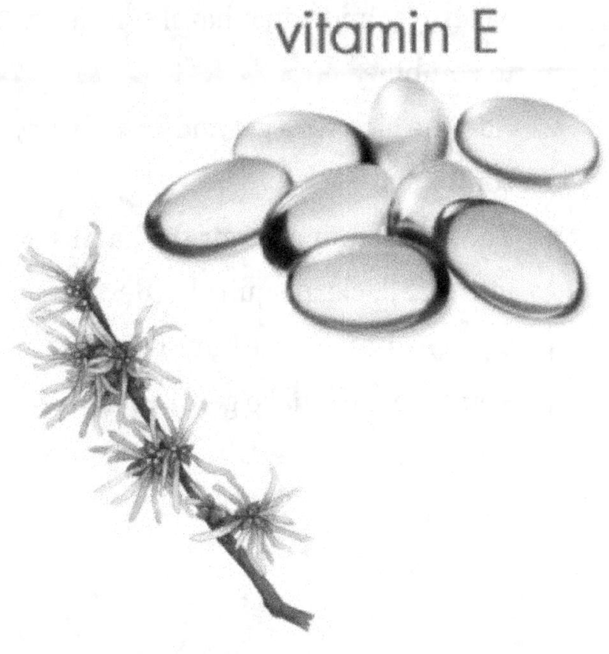

Ingredients:

- ¼ teaspoon vitamin E oil
- 35 drops Germ Destroyer
- 1 tablespoon alcohol-free witch hazel solution
- 1 tablespoon aloe vera gel

Instructions:

1. In a glass bowl, add the vitamin E oil, Germ Destroyer and witch hazel solution and stir to combine.
2. Add the aloe vera gel and mix until well combined.
3. Through a funnel, pour the hand sanitizer into small, clean squirt bottles.
4. Store in a cool place out of direct sunlight.
5. Remember to shake gently before each use.

Vitamin E & Thieves Oil Sanitizer

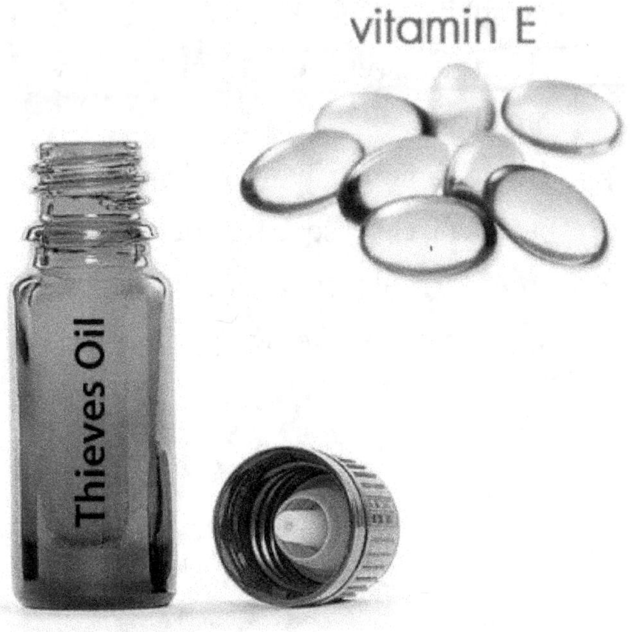

Ingredients:

- ¼ teaspoon vitamin E oil

- 15 drops thieves essential oil blend

- 1/3 cup alcohol-free witch hazel

- 2/3 cup pure aloe vera gel

Instructions:

1. In a glass bowl, add the vitamin E oil, essential oil blend and witch hazel and stir to combine.
2. Add the aloe vera gel and mix until well combined.
3. Through a funnel, pour the hand sanitizer into small, clean squirt bottles.
4. Store in a cool place out of direct sunlight.
5. Remember to shake gently before each use.

Witch Hazel & Peppermint Oil Sanitizer

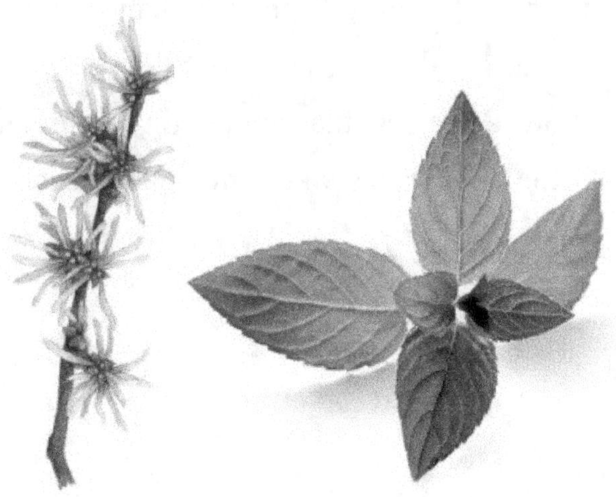

Ingredients:

- 5 drops peppermint essential oil
- 30 drops tea tree oil
- 1½ teaspoons witch hazel
- 1 cup pure aloe vera gel

Instructions:

1. In a glass bowl, add the essential oil, tree oil and witch hazel and witch hazel and stir to combine.
2. Add the aloe vera gel and mix until well combined.
3. Through a funnel, pour the hand sanitizer into small, clean squirt bottles.
4. Store in a cool place out of direct sunlight.
5. Remember to shake gently before each use.

Lemongrass oil & Vodka Sanitizer

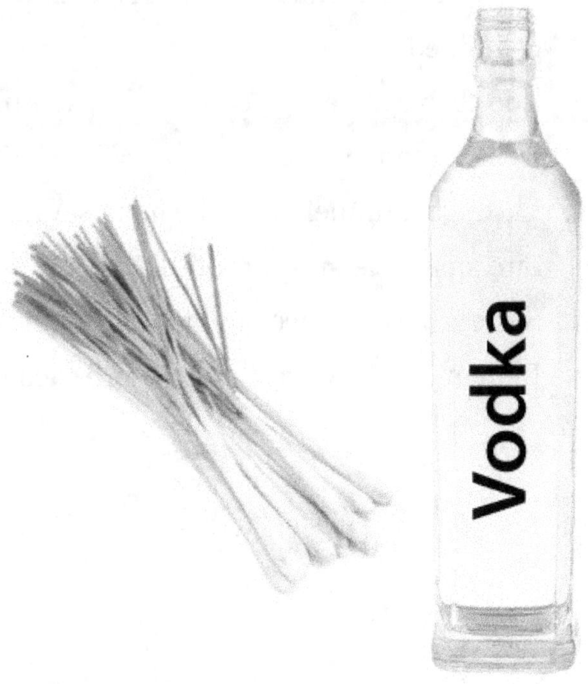

Ingredients:

- ½ cup aloe vera juice
- ¼ cup vodka
- 15-20 drops lemongrass essential oil
- 1 tablespoon vegetable glycerin

Instructions:

1. In a glass bowl, add the aloe vera juice, vodka and essential oil and mix until well combined.

2. Add the vegetable glycerin and mix until well combined.

3. Through a funnel, pour the hand sanitizer into small, clean squirt bottles.

4. Store in a cool place out of direct sunlight.

5. Remember to shake gently before each use.

Apple Cider Vinegar Sanitizer

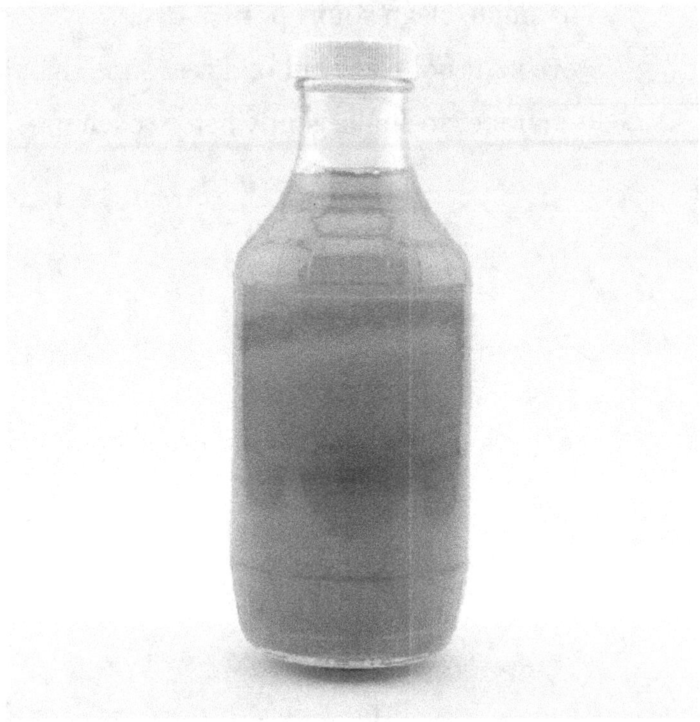

Ingredients:

- ¼ cup apple cider vinegar
- ½ cup aloe vera gel

Instructions:

1. In a glass bowl, add the vinegar and aloe vera gel and mix until well combined.

2. Through a funnel, pour the hand sanitizer into small, clean squirt bottles.

3. Store in a cool place out of direct sunlight.

4. Remember to shake gently before each use.

Witch Hazel & Rosemary Oil Sanitizer

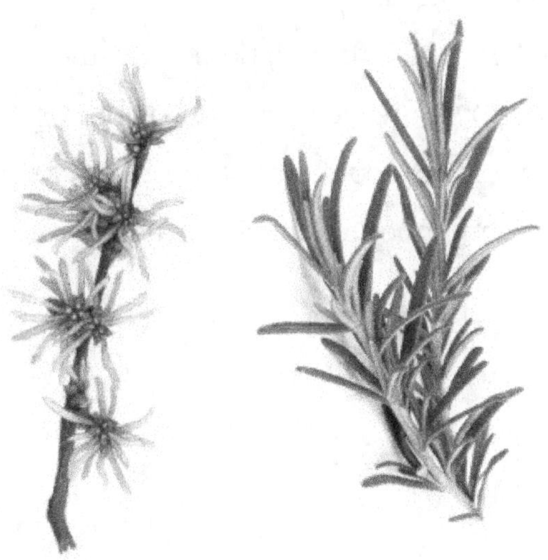

Ingredients:

- 30 drops tea tree oil
- 5-10 drops rosemary essential oil
- 2 tablespoon witch hazel
- 1 cup aloe vera gel

Instructions:

1. In a glass bowl, add the tree oil, essential oil and witch hazel and mix until well combined.
2. Add the aloe vera gel and mix until well combined.
3. Through a funnel, pour the hand sanitizer into small, clean squirt bottles.
4. Store in a cool place out of direct sunlight.
5. Remember to shake gently before each use.

Olivia Holliver's Afterthoughts

Thank you for making it through the end of *Make Your Homemade Hand Sanitizer.*

Your feedback is important to me. It would be greatly appreciated if you could please take a moment to review this book on Amazon so that we could make our next books better.

Blessings!

Olivia Holliver